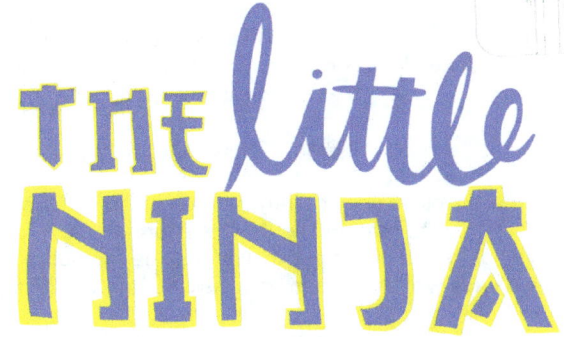

# THE little NINJA

A book about childhood absence epilepsy

**Written by Dr Hayley Lewis**
**Illustrations by James Fox Neville**
**Edited by L-J Ireton**

Bumblebee Books
*London*

BUMBLEBEE PAPERBACK EDITION

Copyright © Dr Hayley Lewis 2021
Illustrations by James Fox Neville

The right of Dr Hayley Lewis to be identified as author of
this work has been asserted in accordance with sections 77 and 78 of the Copyright,
Designs and Patents Act 1988.

All Rights Reserved

No reproduction, copy or transmission of this publication
may be made without written permission.
No paragraph of this publication may be reproduced,
copied or transmitted save with the written permission of the publisher, or in accordance
with the provisions
of the Copyright Act 1956 (as amended).

Any person who commits any unauthorised act in relation to
this publication may be liable to criminal
prosecution and civil claims for damage.

A CIP catalogue record for this title is
available from the British Library.

ISBN: 978-1-83934-138-0

Bumblebee Books is an imprint of
Olympia Publishers.

First Published in 2021

Bumblebee Books
Tallis House
2 Tallis Street
London
EC4Y 0AB

Printed in Great Britain

www.olympiapublishers.com

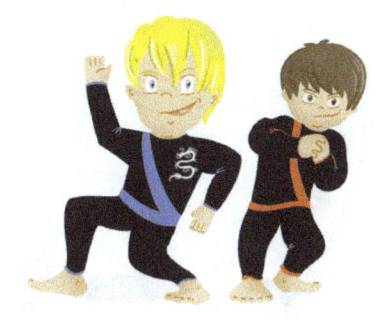

**For Jago and Saxon**

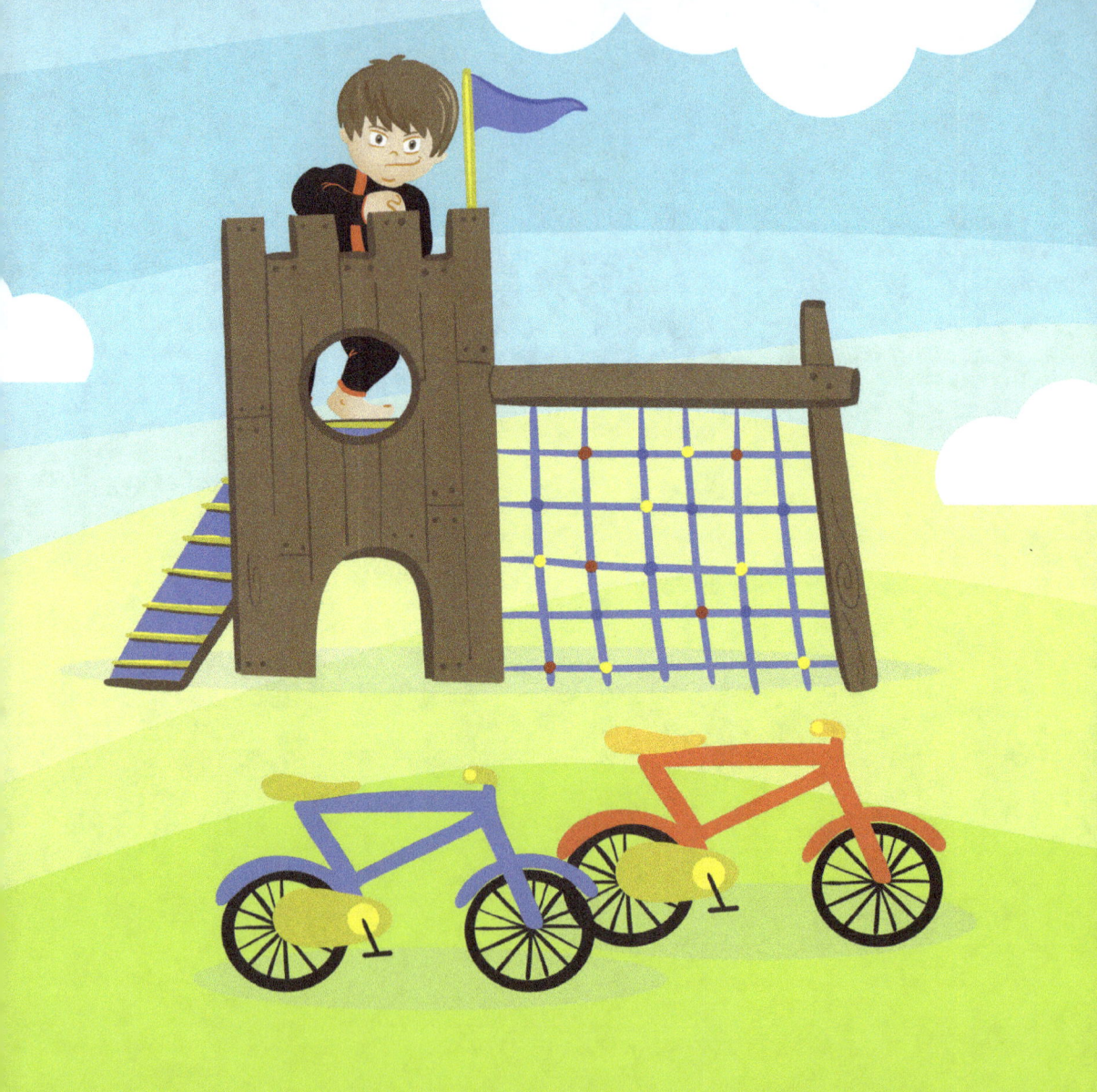

Meet The Little Ninja and his sidekick, Younger Bro.
They love to climb and trampoline. They're always on the go.

Wearing ninja outfits, one in red and one in blue,
they run and fight and hide. They do all things ninjas do.

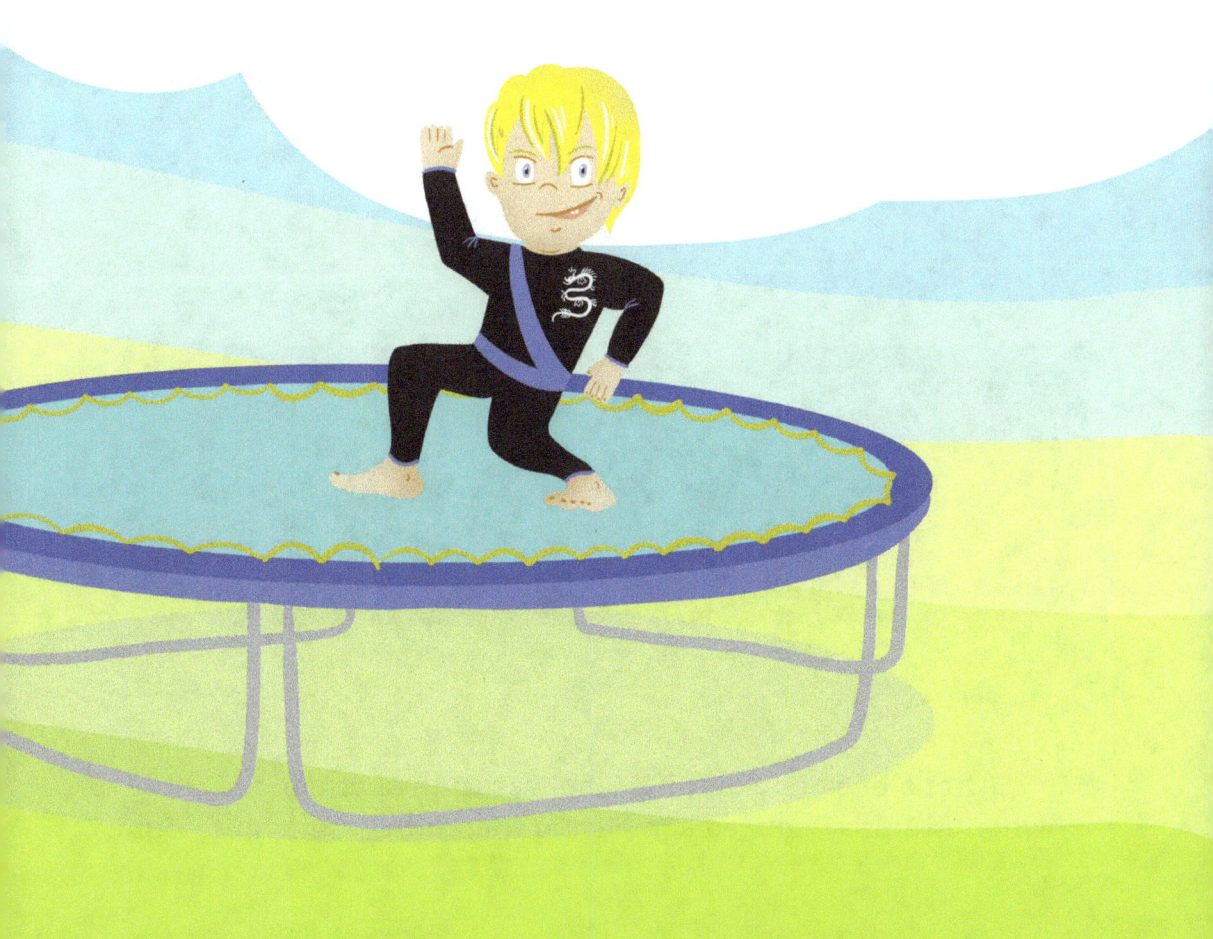

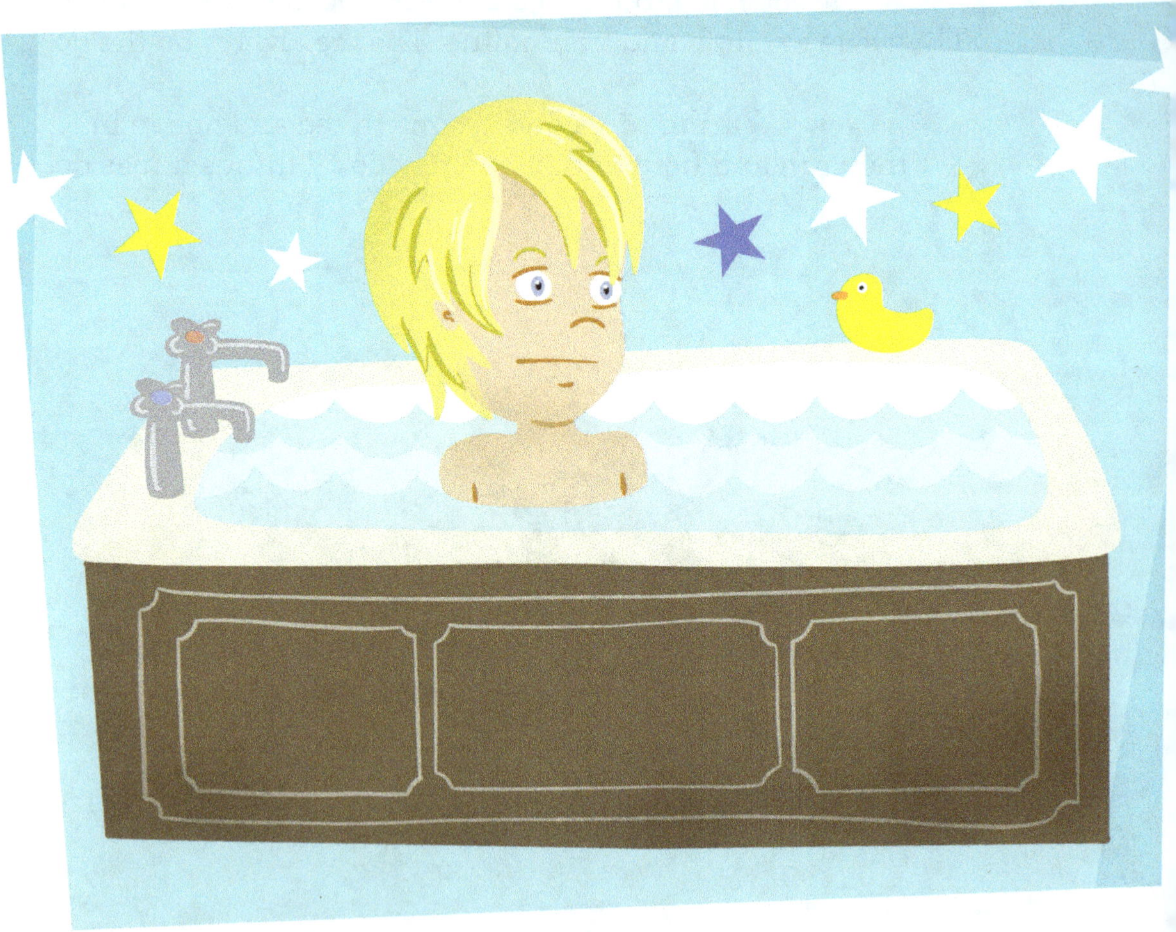

After a busy day of ninjas, he was in the bath one night,
when Mummy noticed something that didn't seem quite right.

The Little Ninja stopped and stared off into space,
he lost his cheeky smile and he had a blank face.

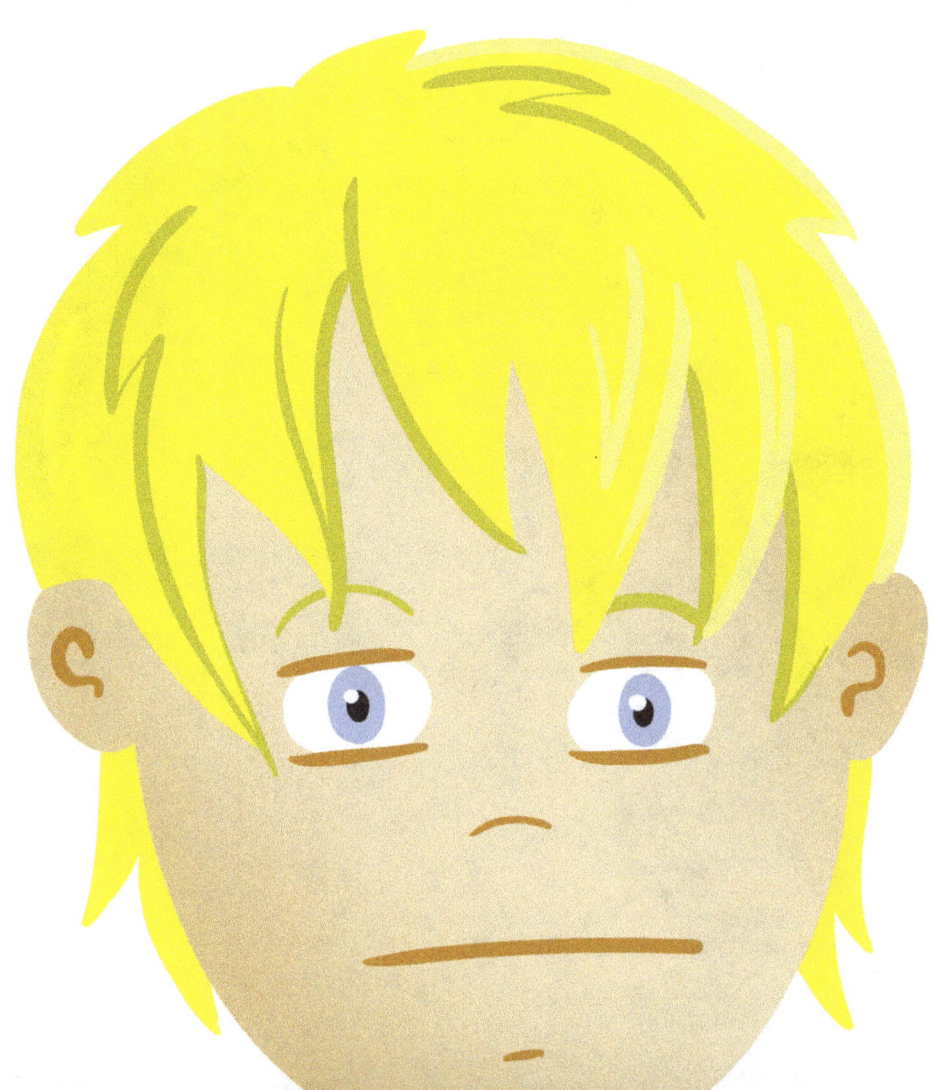

They went to the hospital and to the **Children's Ward**.
There were so many toys! The Little Ninja wasn't bored.

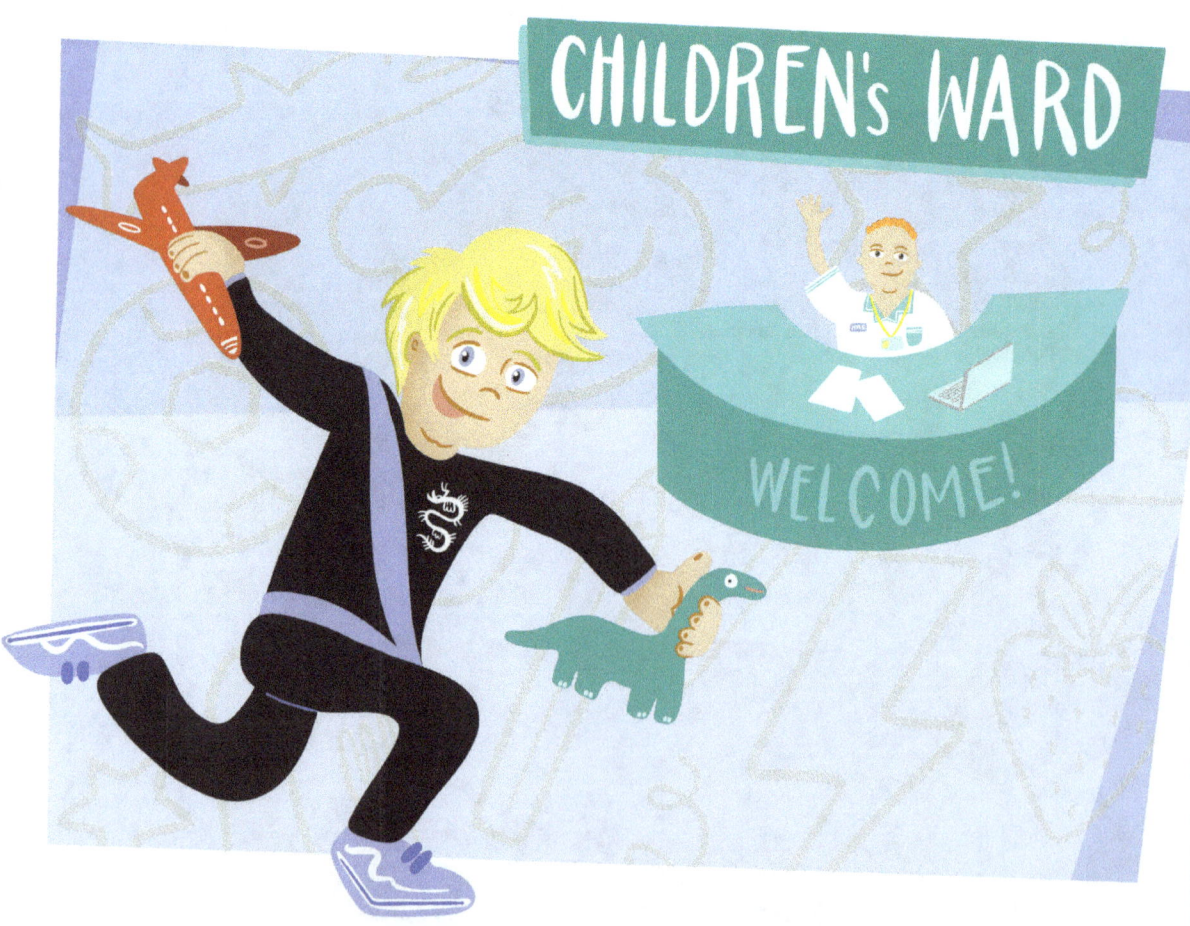

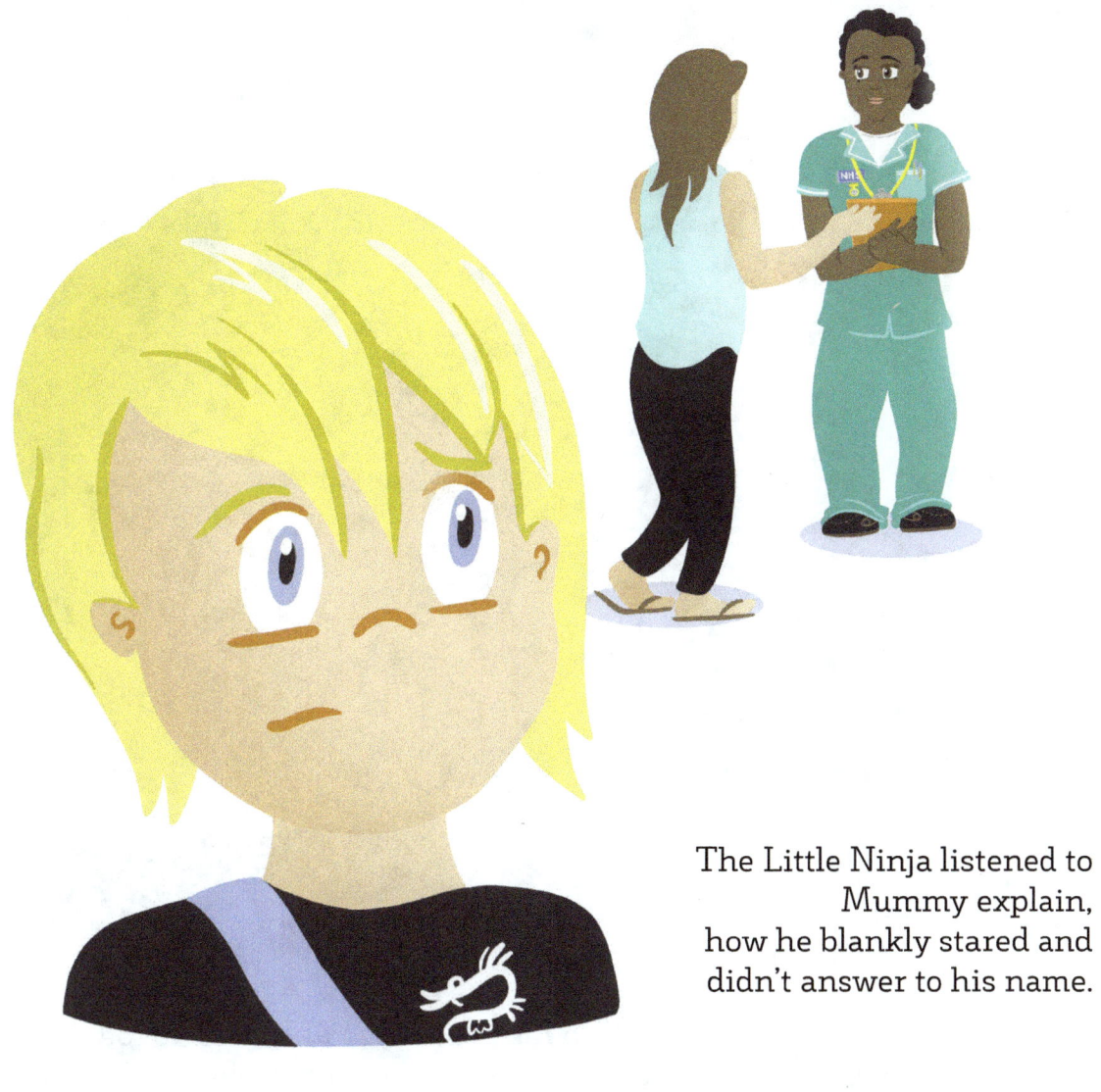

The Little Ninja listened to Mummy explain, how he blankly stared and didn't answer to his name.

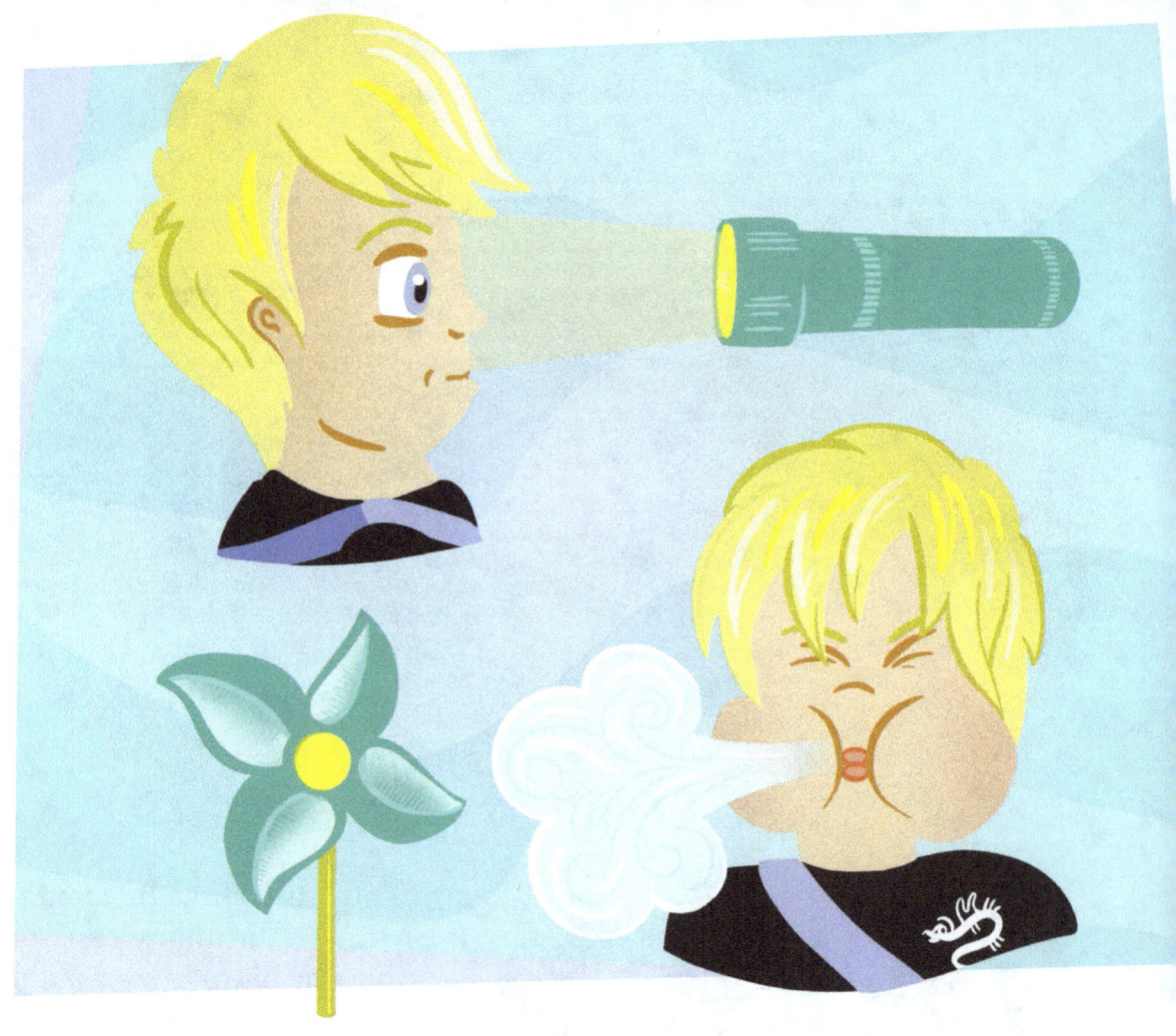

They shined a light into his eyes. He walked heel to toe.
They found a paper windmill and he was told to blow and blow.

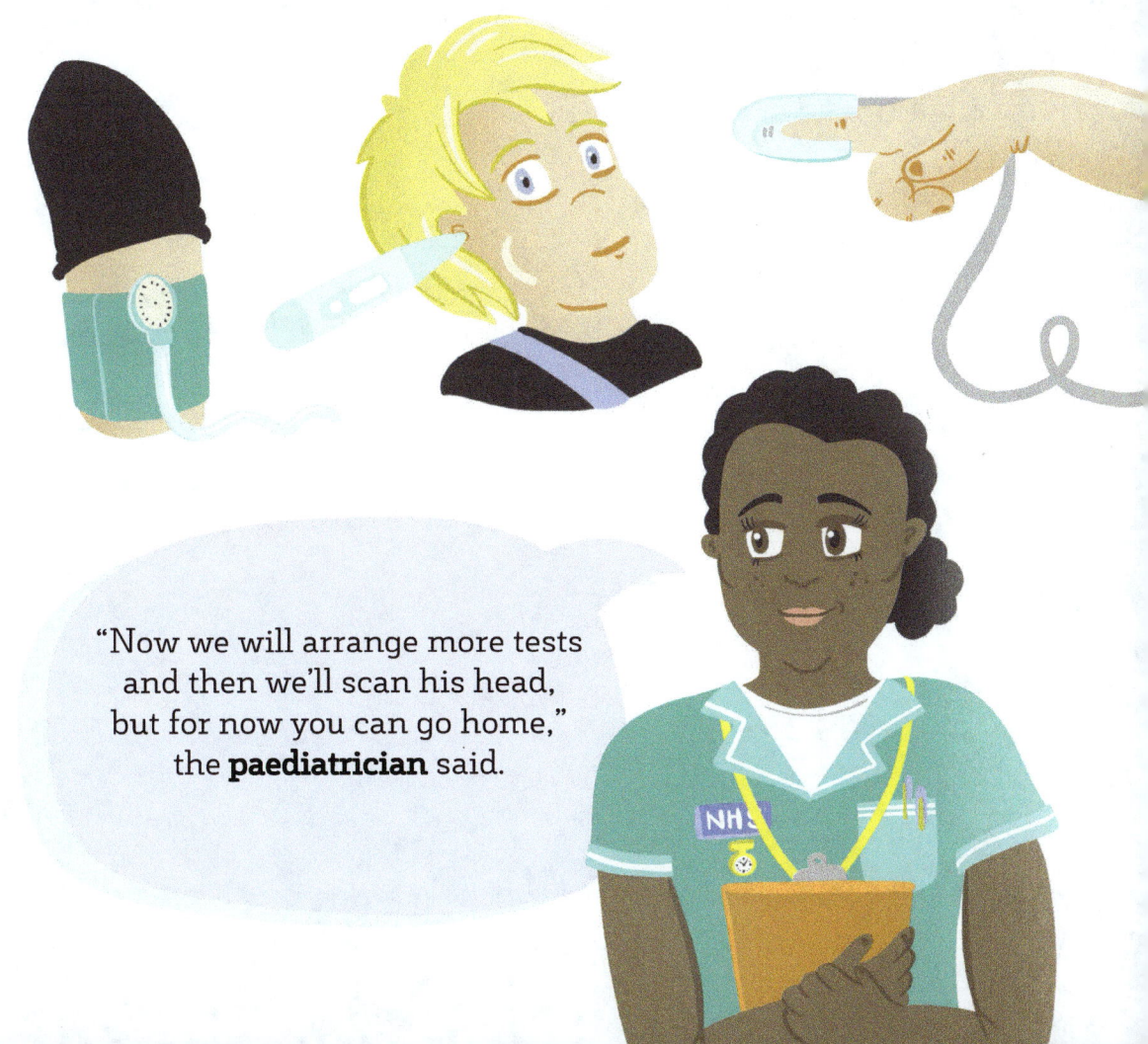

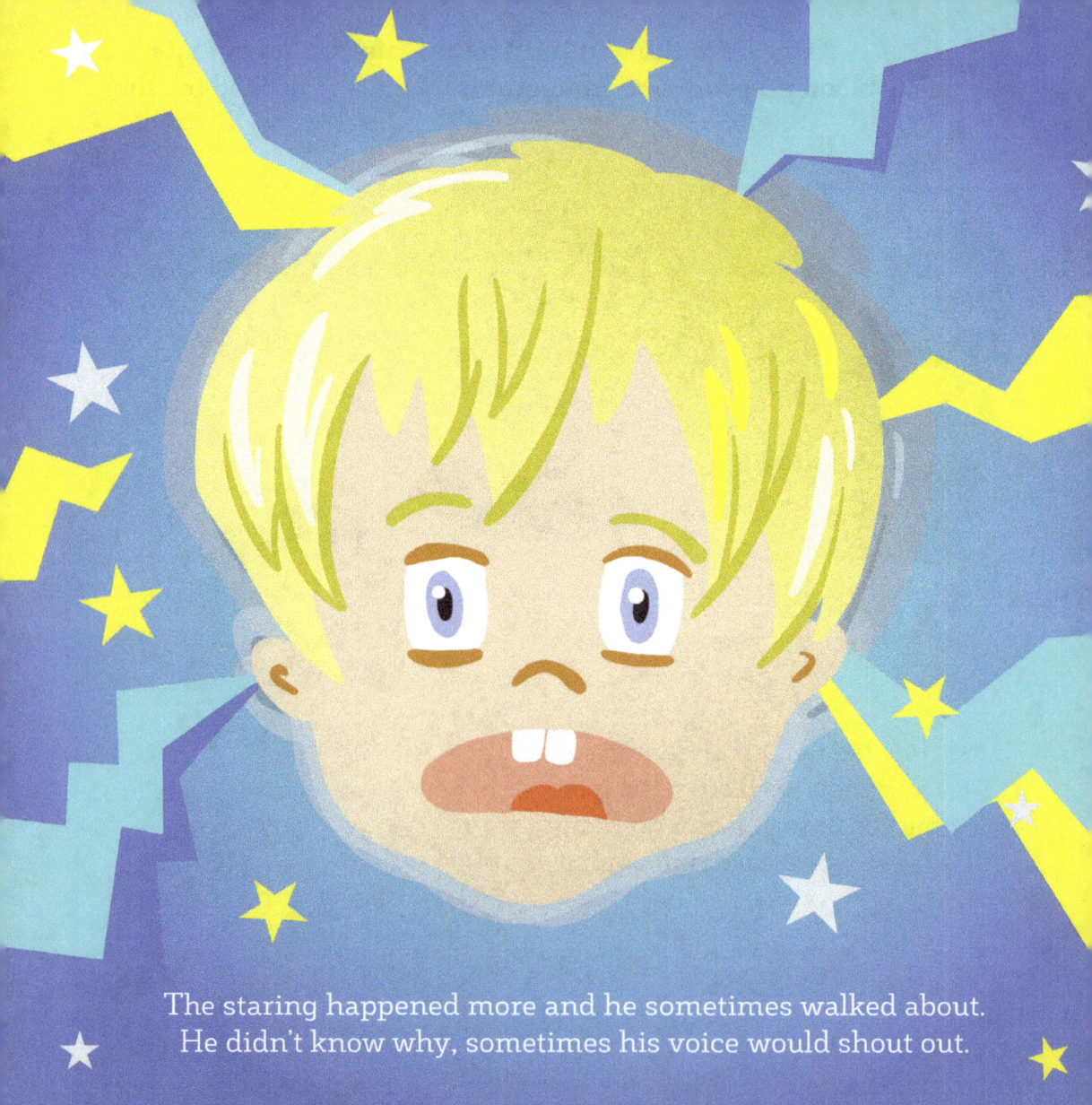

The staring happened more and he sometimes walked about.
He didn't know why, sometimes his voice would shout out.

One day in music class he was giving the maracas a good shake.
Then he found himself elsewhere — like sleepwalking, and now awake.

At school his friends asked questions,

"Why do you wander, shout and stare?"

"I don't know,"

The Little Ninja said,

"I'm completely unaware."

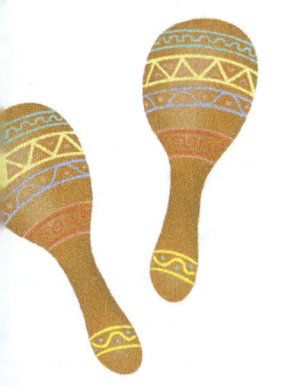
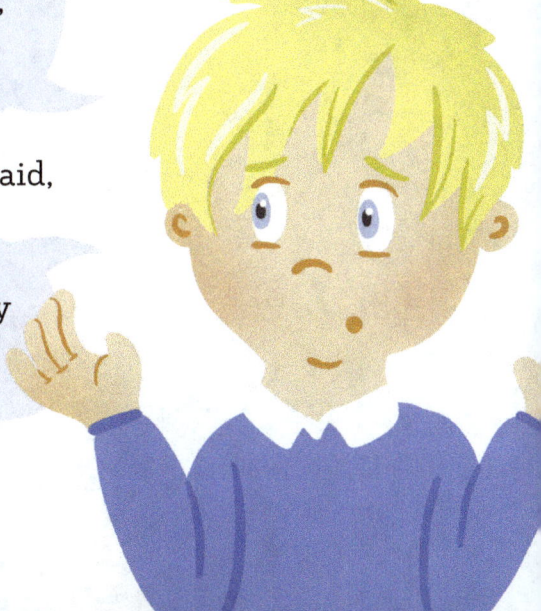

Daddy took him for a special test, it was called an **EEG**.
He wore a silly hat to measure his brain's electricity.

He had to sit still on a chair, just his teddy and himself.
Daddy laughed and told him, "You look like Santa's elf!"

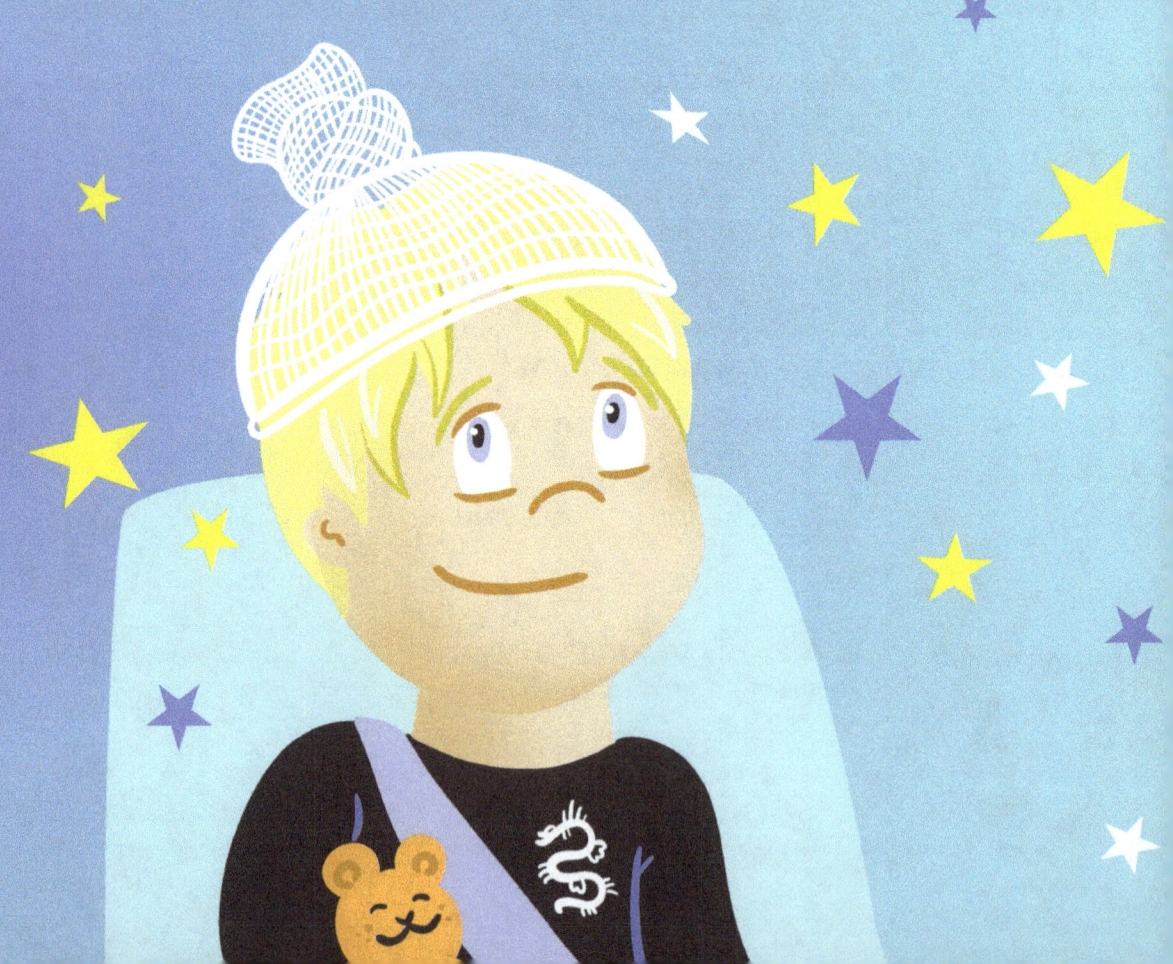

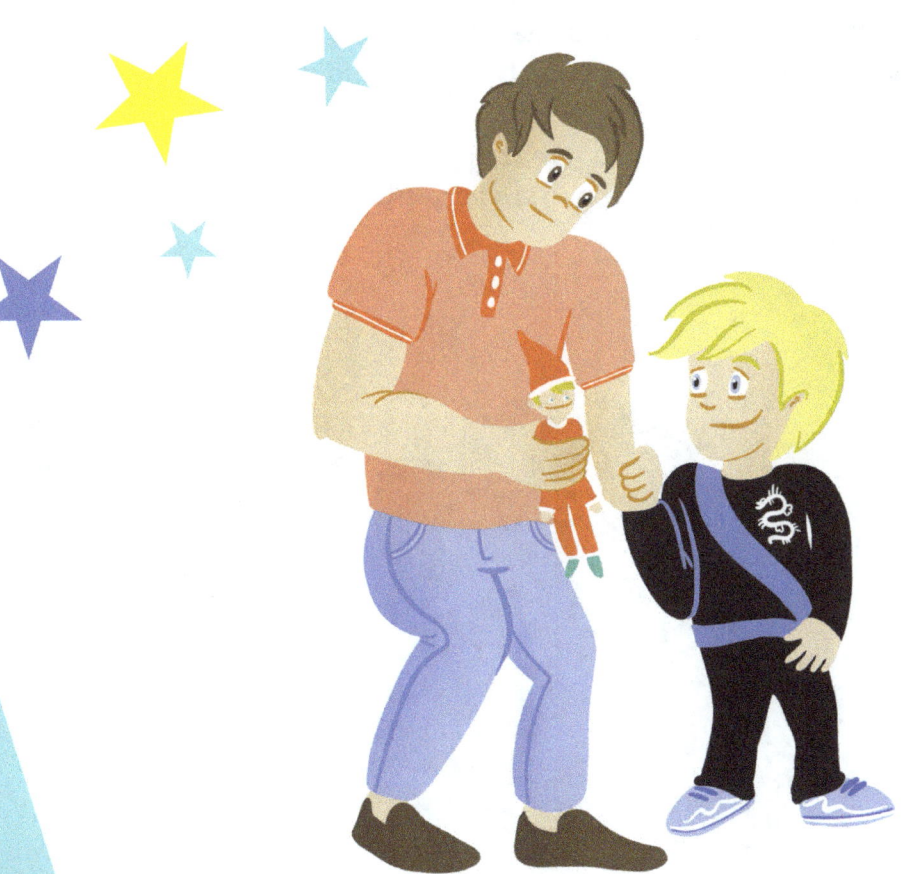

The test did not take long and for being a good boy,
Daddy took him to the shop and bought him an elf toy.

The **CT scan** was easy, he just had to lie still.
But staying still was not exactly his top ninja skill!

Mummy stood right by him, wearing an apron made of lead,
whilst he moved through the 'giant doughnut'
taking pictures of his head.

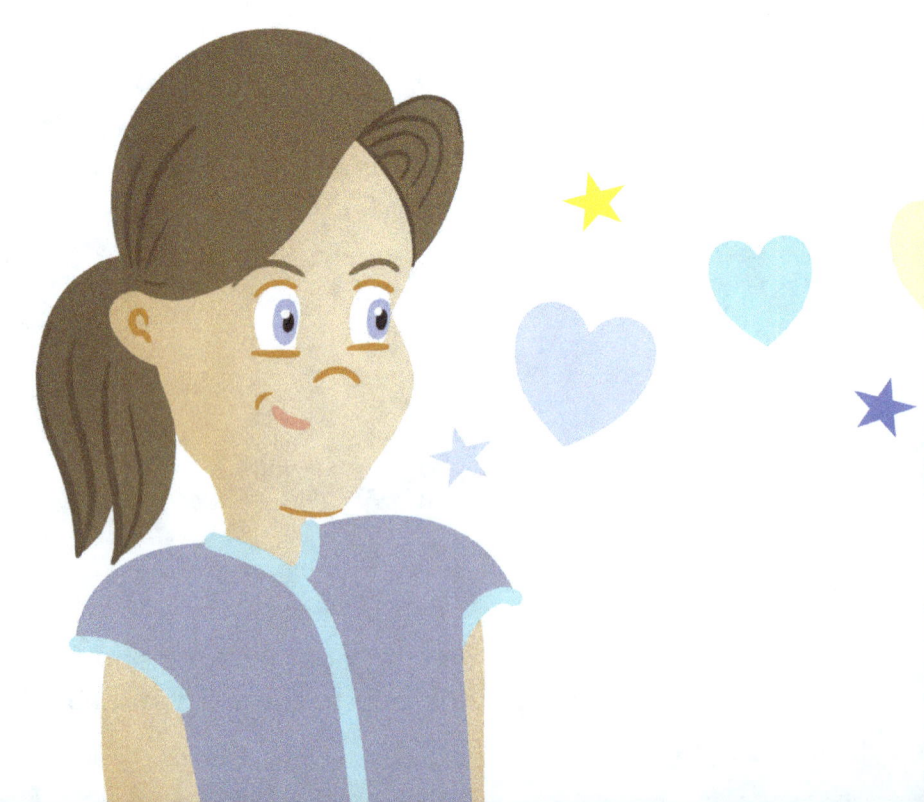

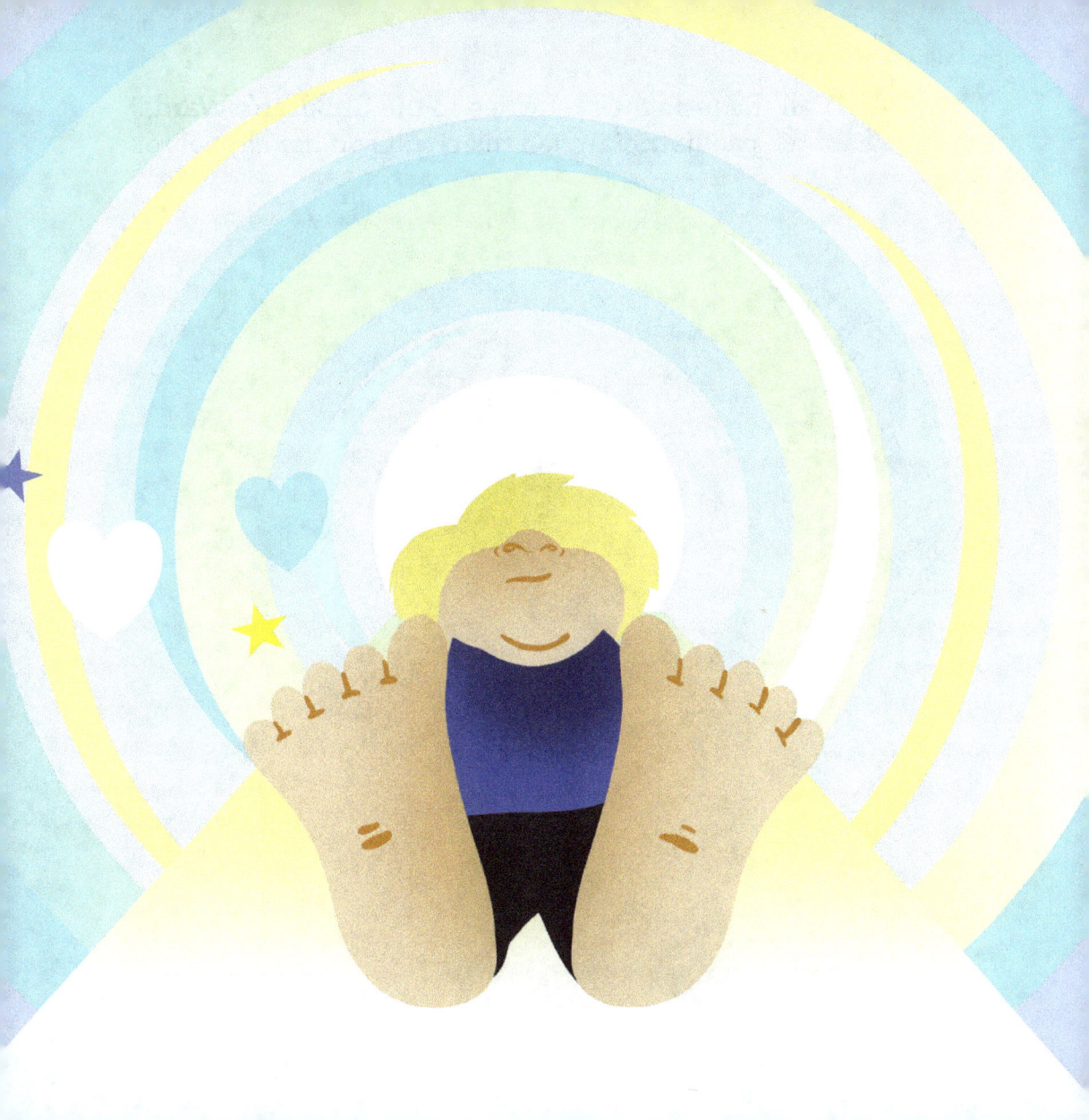

After all the tests they returned to the **Children's Ward**, where his **paediatrician** had his results on her clipboard.

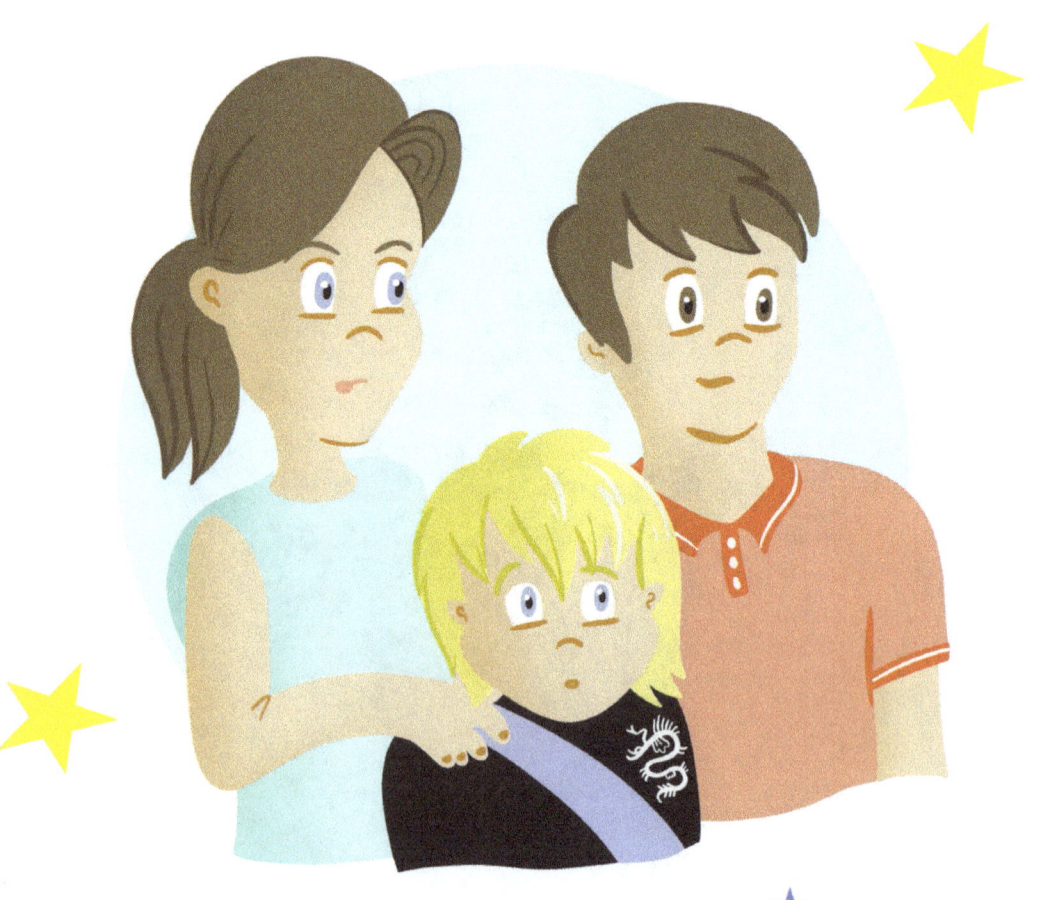

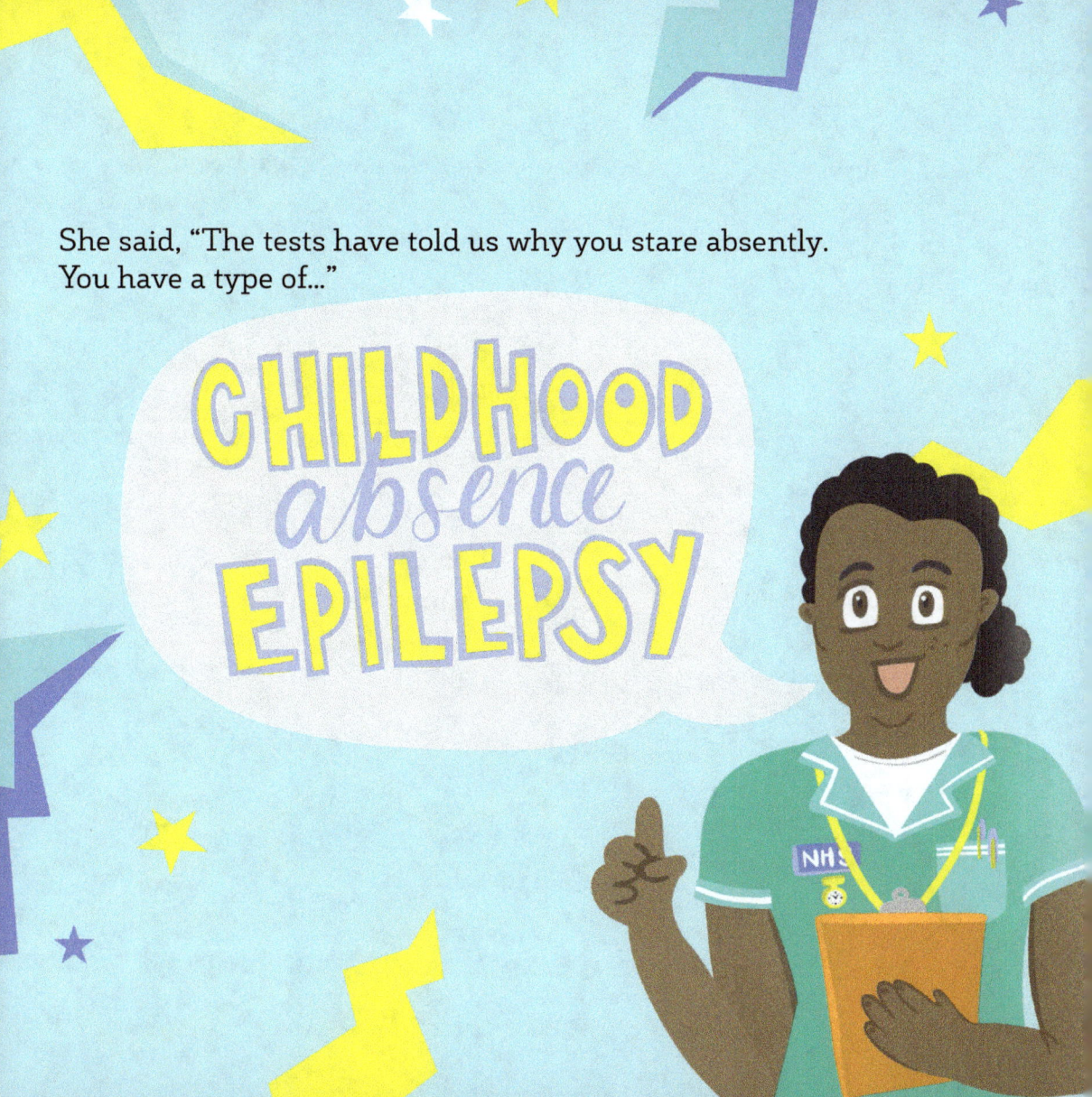

"What is that?" he asked and she went on to explain,
"It's like there's extra electricity running through your brain."

"With medicine we can keep the epilepsy at bay,
and it is extremely likely you will grow out of it one day."

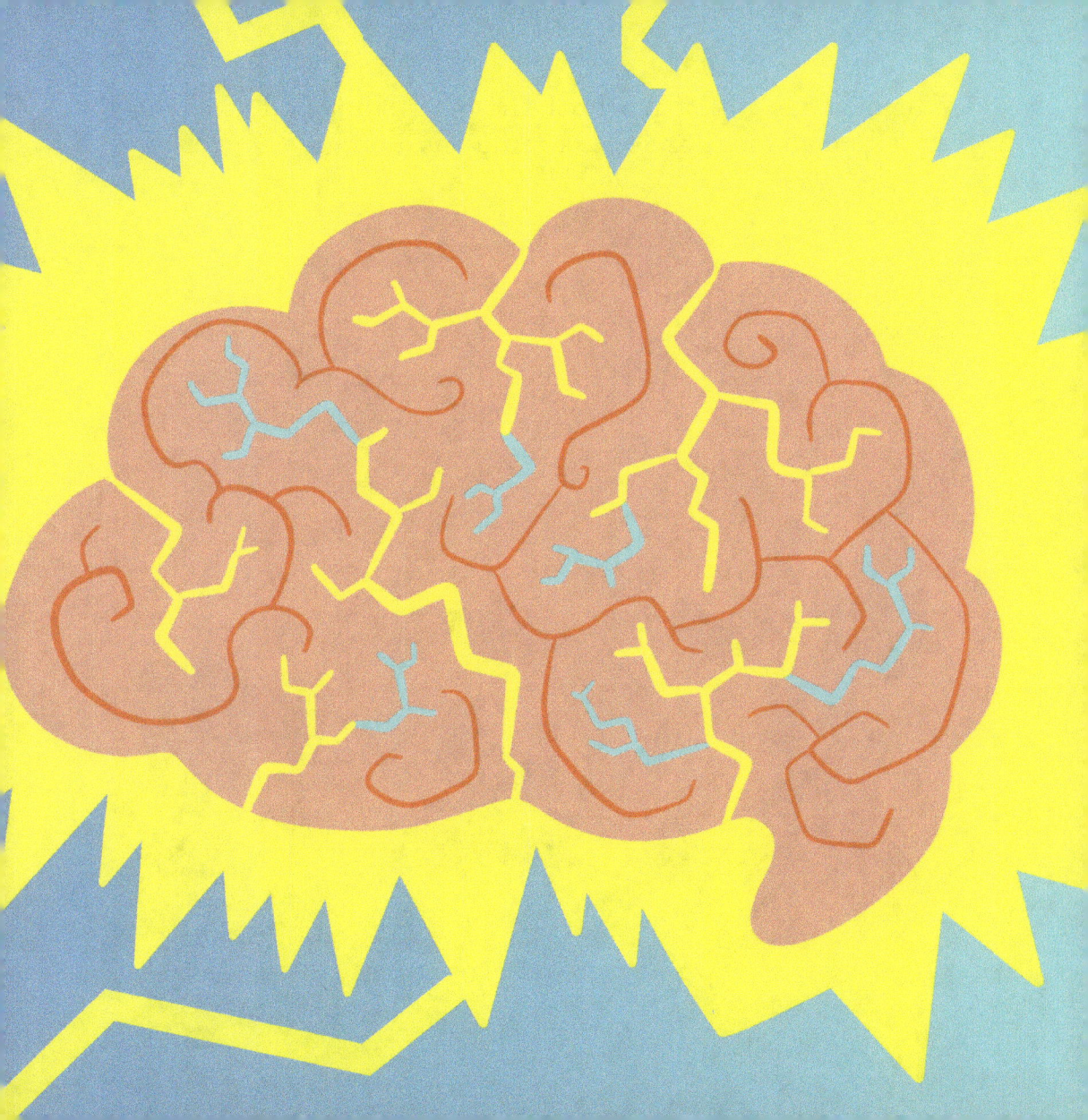

The next day whilst at school The Little Ninja had no shame, in telling all his friends his staring has a name.

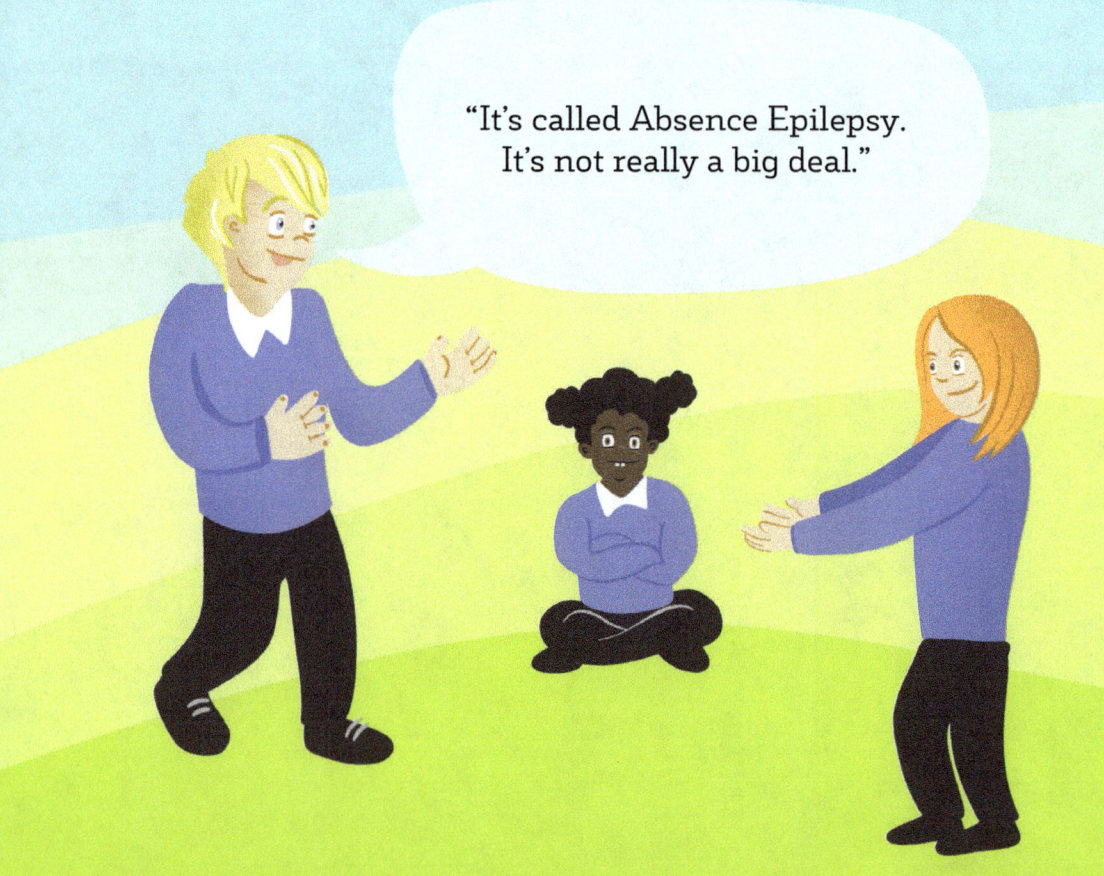

"It's called Absence Epilepsy. It's not really a big deal."

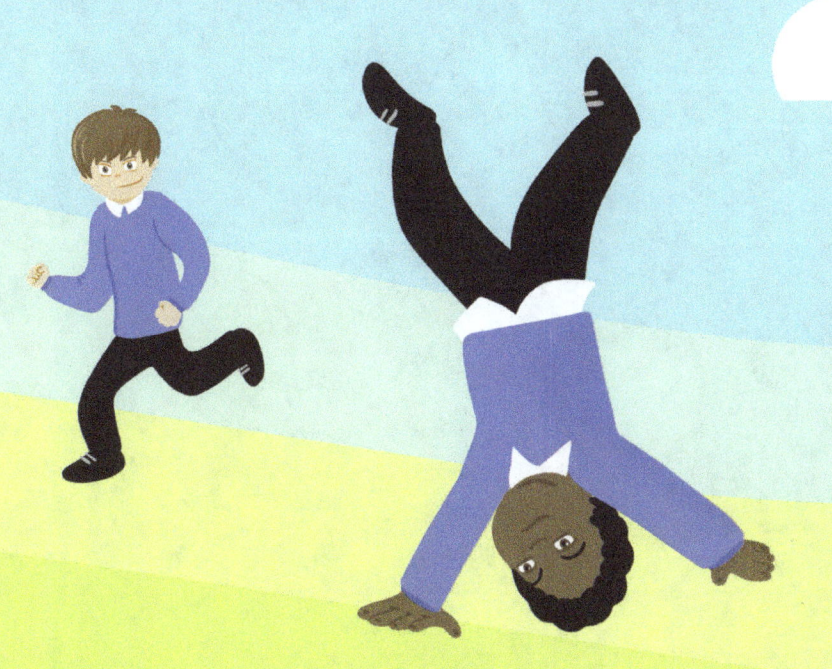

And off they ran to play and skip, tumble and cartwheel.

The Little Ninja took his medicine every day and night.
His staring into space vanished out of sight.

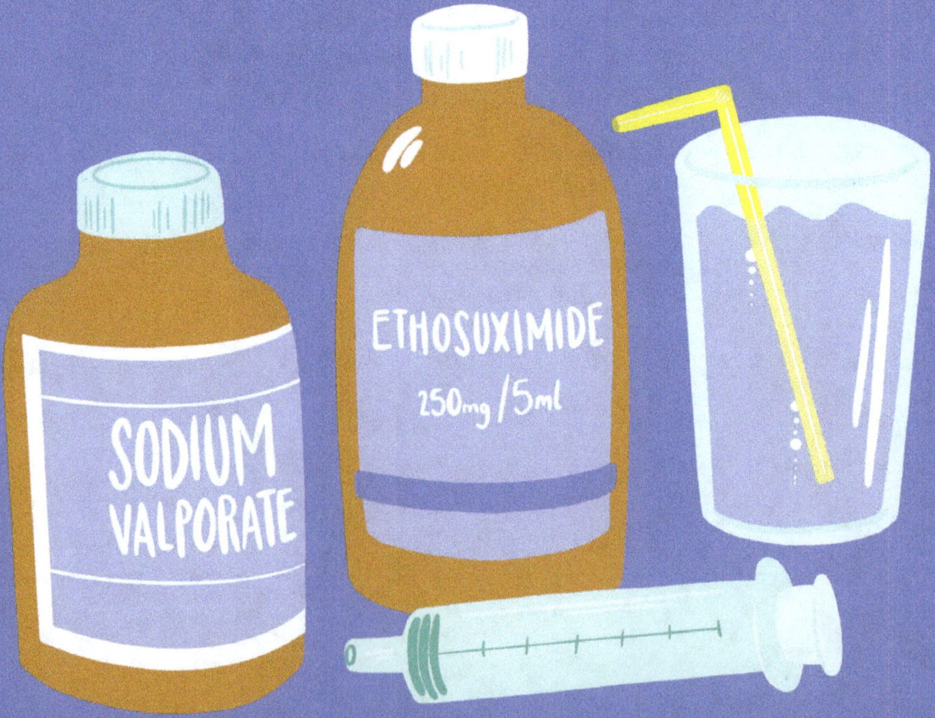

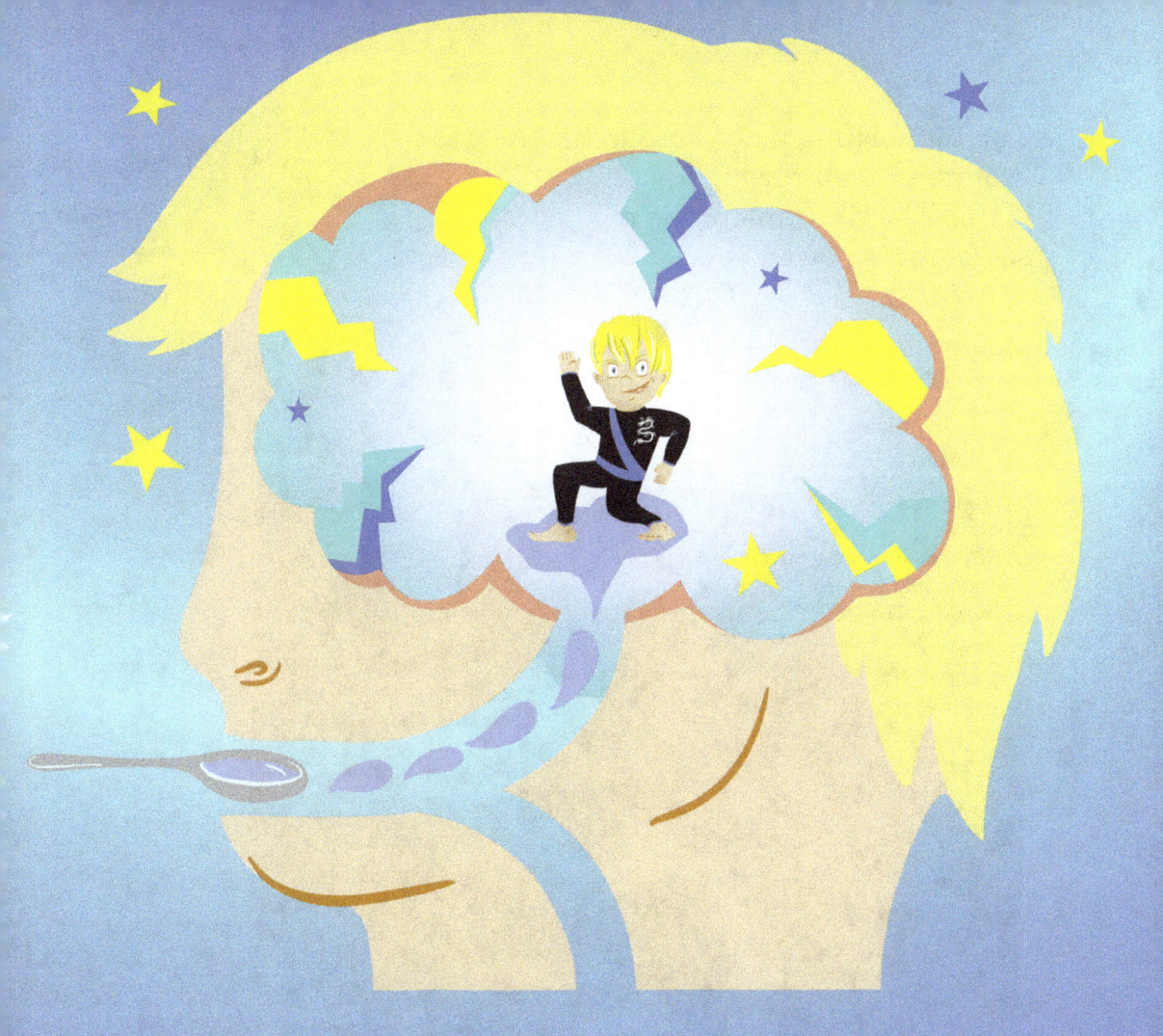

"Do I still have epilepsy?" The Little Ninja asked one day.
Mummy replied, "Yes, it's the medicine keeping it away".

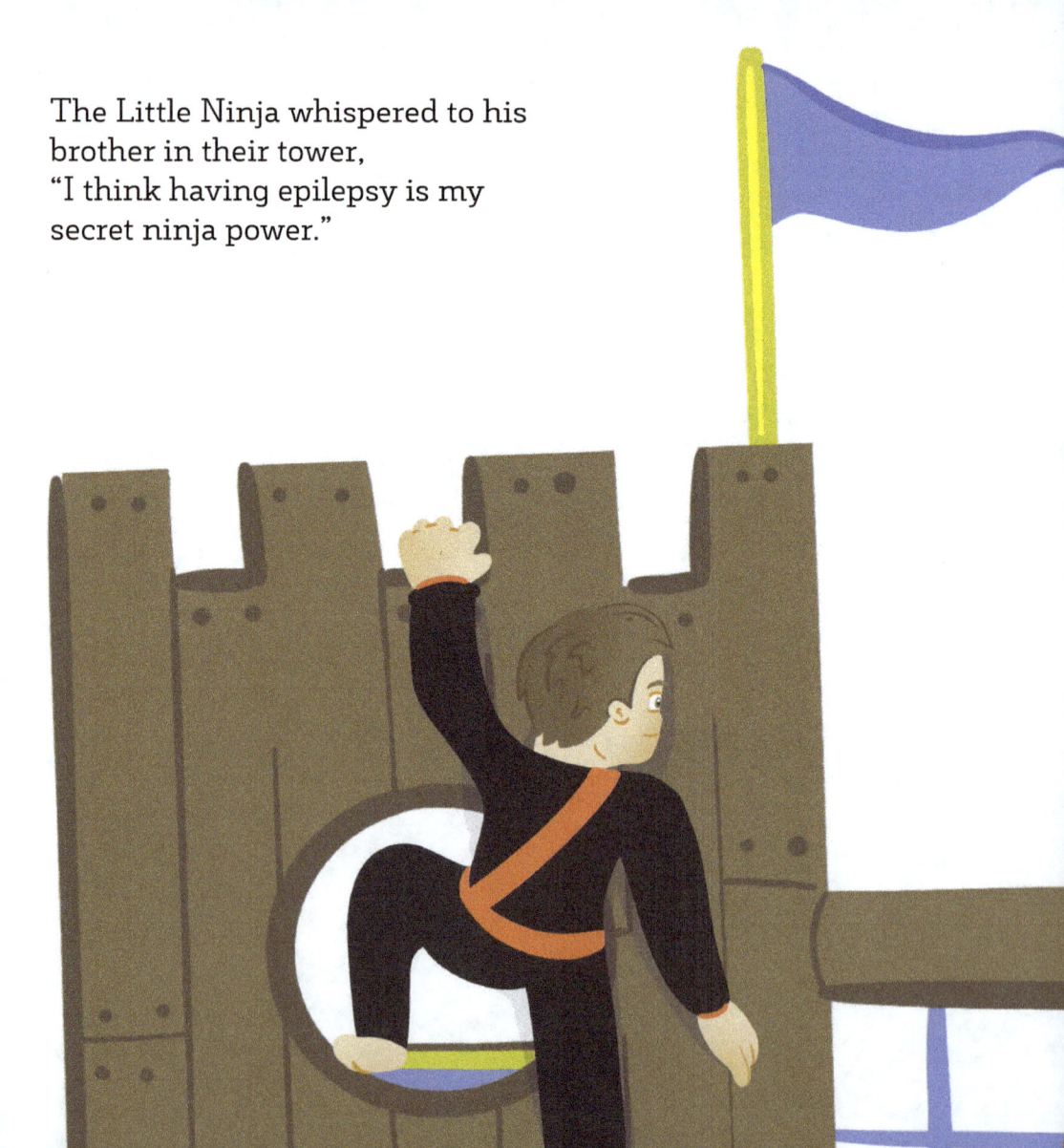

The Little Ninja whispered to his brother in their tower,
"I think having epilepsy is my secret ninja power."

"I'm the only one, none of my friends have **epilepsy**,
It helps to make me special, it makes me ME!"

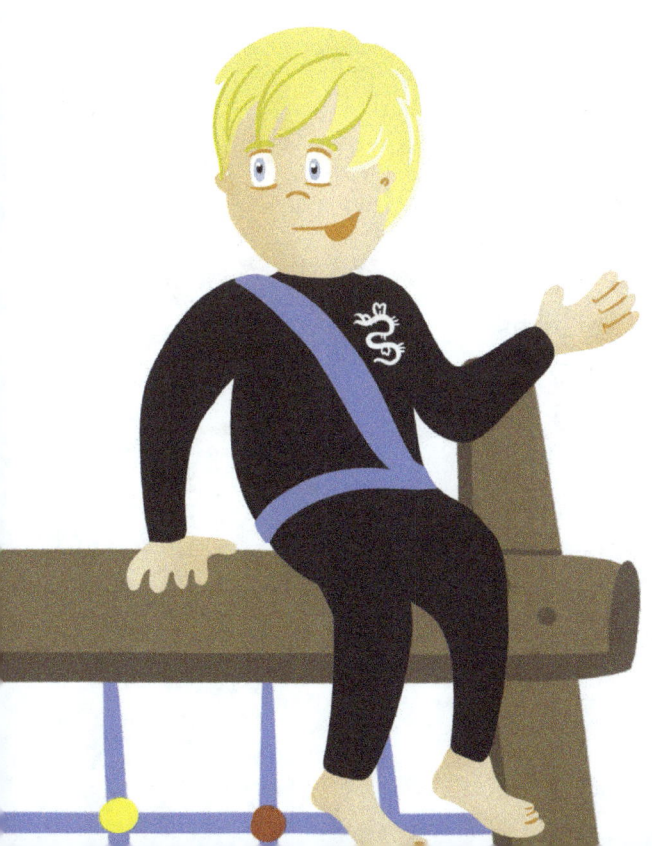

# Glossary

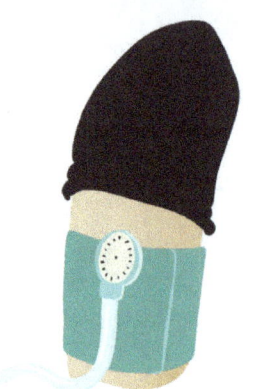

**Blood Pressure:** This is a measurement of the pressure in arteries (blood tubes in the body). It is measured by placing a cuff around the upper arm which slowly tightens and loosens again.

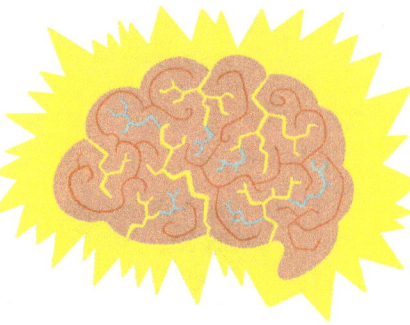

**Childhood Absence Epilepsy:** Epilepsy is when the brain has sudden bursts of extra electricity causing a seizure or fit. There are lots of different types of epilepsy causing different types of seizures. In Childhood Absence Epilepsy the seizures are usually brief and look like staring. It starts in childhood and most children grow out of it.

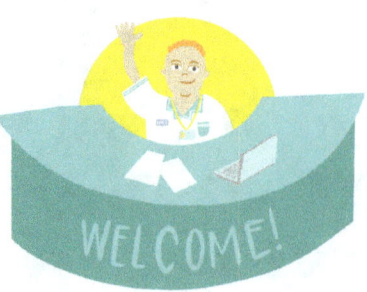

**Children's Ward:** Rooms in the hospital are called wards. The Children's Ward is the area of the hospital which cares for children.

**CT Scan (Computed Tomography Scan):** This is a test to look inside the body using X-rays. The CT scanner machine has a bed which moves slowly through a large ring taking photographs of inside the body. People who are nearby usually wear a heavy lead apron because this protects them from the X-rays.

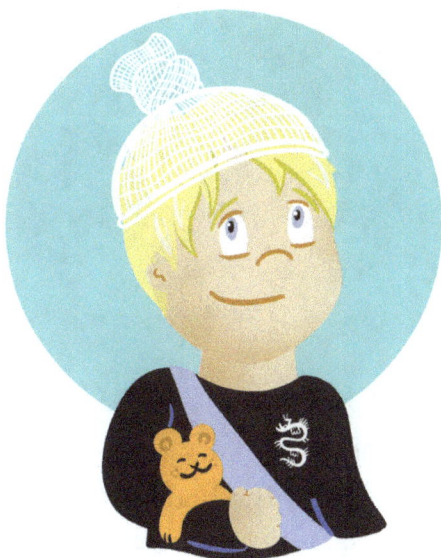

**EEG (Electroencephalogram):** This is a special test to measure the brain's activity. Wires are placed on the head to measure the electricity in the brain and a computer records this.

**Paediatrician:** A doctor who treats and looks after children.

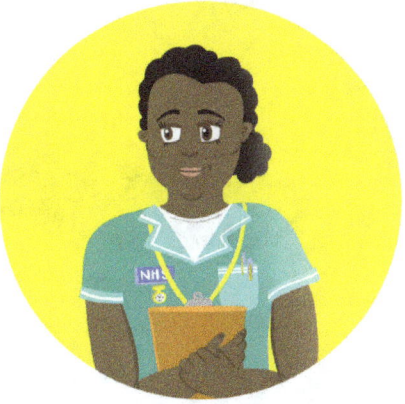

**Pulse:** This tells the doctor how the heart is beating and can be felt at different places in the body, usually the wrist. Sometimes doctors and nurses use a small machine placed on the finger, which looks like a peg, to measure a pulse. The machine also tells them how much oxygen is in the blood.

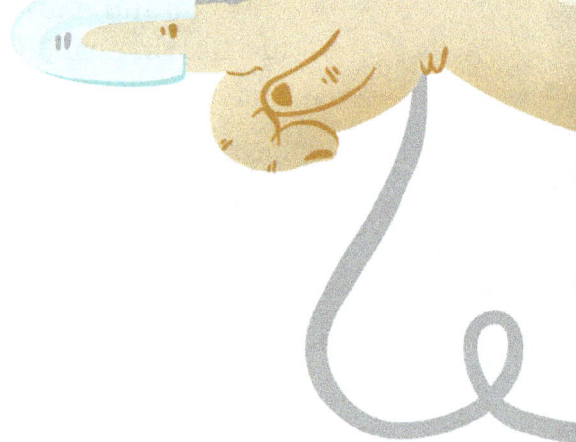

**Temperature:** This is a measurement of how hot or cold the body is. It is measured with a thermometer, which is placed inside the mouth or ear.

## About the Author

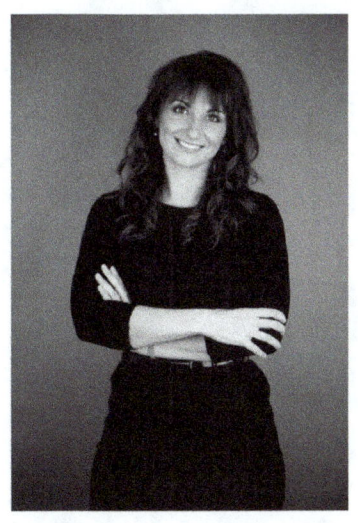

Dr Hayley Lewis is a Cheshire-based NHS GP and mother to two very active little boys. When her eldest son was diagnosed with childhood absence epilepsy, she felt inspired to write a book to help explain the condition to her son, his friends and to also reassure children who were facing the same diagnosis.

www.ingramcontent.com/pod-product-compliance
Lightning Source LLC
LaVergne TN
LVHW081526060526
838200LV00044B/2015